MRSA Infection in Home Care

By Sharon C Kelly, Registered Nurse

MRSA in Homecare ● What is an Infection? ● Definition of MRSA ● Signs and Symptoms of MRSA ● Where Does MRSA Live and Grow? ● How is MRSA Spread? ● Standard Precautions ● Proper Handwashing Technique ● Alcohol Based Hand Gels ● Gloving and Gowning ● Treatment of MRSA ● MRS A on Household S urfac es ● How to Handle Spills ● MRSA and Housekeeping ● MRSA and Urinary Tract Infection ● MRSA and Pneumonia ● Conclusion

MRSA IN HOME CARE

Are you caring for someone in their home? If you are, you are among a growing number of health care workers. The demand for home care aids and home care services is increasing due to the growing number of older adults and chronically ill people living in their own home. The information that I am going to share with you in this book about MRSA infection in home care is something that you should be acutely aware of as you care for your patients. Not only should you be knowledgeable for your patient's protection, but for your own protection as well.

MRSA infection among home care patients in the community is now becoming widespread and anyone can be at risk. The MRSA bacterium (germ) was at one time seen only in hospitals and nursing homes but now it is being seen in increasing numbers in the homecare setting. Don't ever underestimate the capabilities of this superbug, as it is now called, and its capacity to cause great harm. You are caring for someone who is compromised in some way and therefore is more susceptible to what this germ can do, which is to cause an infection.

Most people who get MRSA get a skin infection. This could be a wound or a surgical site. However, MRSA infections can also occur on the skin where there is no break. It can occur anywhere on a person's body. MRSA is widespread and can be spread by close skin to skin contact, cuts and abrasions, contaminated surfaces and poor hygiene.

This book is meant to be a handy guide for you as you go about your daily tasks in caring for your patient. Each person you care for is different and no two jobs will be alike. However, there are some very important commonalities. These commonalities are what I would like to focus on because they are simple steps you can take in the care of all your patients to help curtail the spread of MRSA in the home care setting. Caring for other people can be challenging, but you will heap great rewards. Remember, you are helping someone to stay in their home and be independent for as long as possible. How long a person is able to stay at home could depend on the care you give them. You have an awesome responsibility. Because MRSA is not just in the hospital or nursing home setting any more, patients, family and caregivers need to be able to recognize the sources of infection and ways to prevent infections from happening. The best way to protect those being cared for in the home is to teach you, the caregiver, so you can teach your patients and their families how the infectious process works.

WHAT IS AN INFECTION?

A simple explanation is that an infection is a growth of harmful microscopic organisms or germs, in the body. You need to remember, however, that just because there is a pathogen or germ present in someone's body that an infection will automatically occur. This is not always true because an infection must occur in a cycle and the cycle depends on all elements in the cycle to be present. One way to describe this cycle is to picture a chain with 6 links all linked together. This chain is a way of explaining how a disease can be spread from one person to another. Every one of the links that make up the chain must be intact for an infection to occur. What are these six links?

The first link in the chain is a bug or germ that causes disease. For example, this could be a virus that causes the flu or maybe a bacterium that causes a sore throat or MRSA in a wound.

The second link in the chain is the place where this virus or bacterium can live and grow. This is someplace where the bug hides. Microorganisms or pathogens grow best in warm, dark, and moist places. Some examples of this in the human body are lungs, blood, large intestine and skin.

The third link in this chain is how these bugs escape from where they are living and growing. This can happen when one of the infected person's body openings lets the bug escape. This could be by a cough, or through pus or drainage from a wound infection, or through feces from the GI tract.

The fourth link in the chain of infection is how this germ travels from one person to another. This happens through the air, or by touching an infected persons secretions or by touching something that has been contaminated by the infected person such as clothing, bedrail, etc.

The fifth link is how the pathogen gets into an uninfected person's body. This of course, is through the persons' body openings. This can occur through the nose, mouth or any mucous membrane or a cut in the skin. Once the pathogen finds an uninfected person, such as a caregiver like you, it can make you sick because you are susceptible. This means you are not already infected with that particular disease.

However, if one of the above links is broken, then the spread of infection is stopped. If you use good infection control practices, you can stop the germ from entering your body. You will hear over and over again that the best way to stop the spread of infection, or break the chain, is through proper hand hygiene.

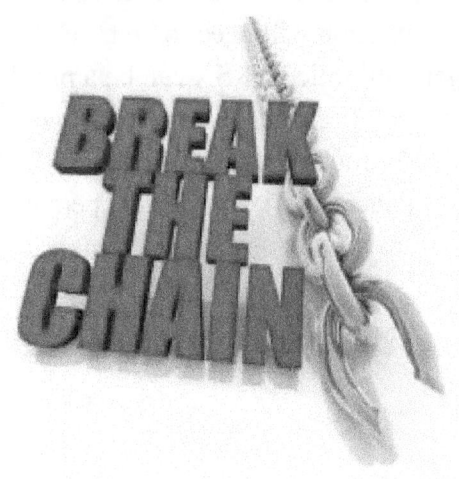

DEFINITION OF MRSA

MRSA stands for Methicillin Resistant Staphylococcus aureus. Let's begin by defining Staph aureus or Staph. Staph is a bacterium (germ) that is carried on the skin or in the nasal passages of many healthy individuals and usually causes no problems. Methicillin resistant means that the Staph bacterium is resistant to the drug Methicillin and other antibiotics related to Methicillin. These powerful antibiotics are related to penicillin which used to be used to treat a staph infection. So what this means is the infection will need to be treated with a different type and even stronger antibiotic. MRSA can be a problem for those patients that you are caring for because they are usually older adults or people with compromised immune systems. If a person's skin is damaged in any way, the Staph bacterium can enter the person thru the injury and cause anywhere from mild to severe problems.

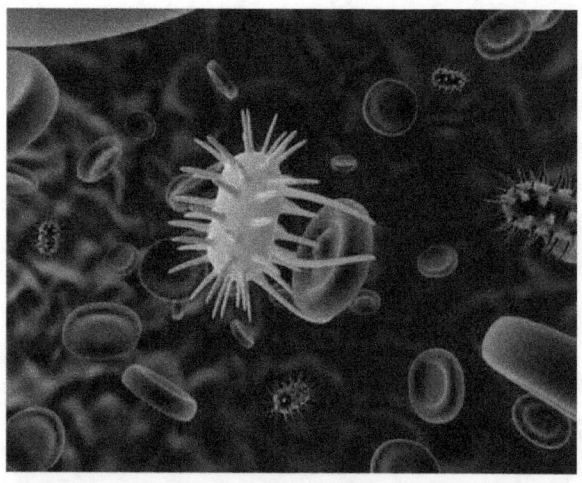

SIGNS AND SYMPTOMS OF MRSA

 In the community, most MRSA infections are skin infections. A skin infection is usually characterized by a lump or bump that is tender and may even be draining some pus. It usually will become more tender, red and swollen as time goes on. Sometimes it might even look like a spider bite. The patient may also experience pain and fever.

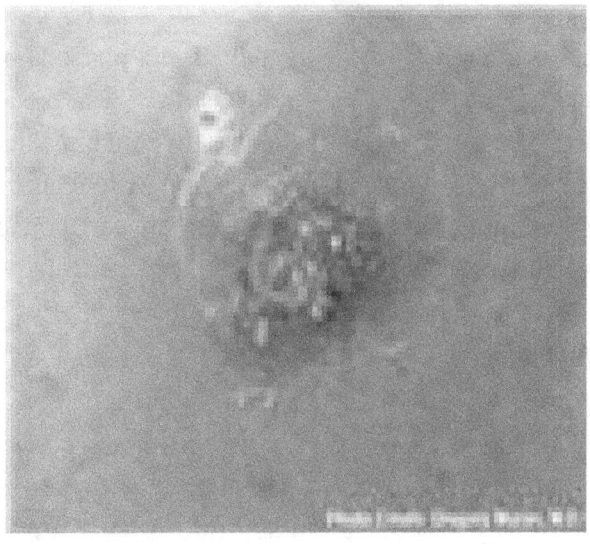

WHERE DOES MRSA LIVE & GROW?

Remember the second link in the chain is that the germ needs a place to live and grow. As we said before, the best places for microorganisms to grow are warm, dark and moist and these places in the body include the nose, skin, lungs, blood and large intestine.

HOW IS MRSA SPREAD?

MRSA is almost always spread by direct physical contact and through the air e.g. coughing. However, it can also be spread through indirect contact. The direct way of spread is by touching an infected person who has MRSA on his skin. Spreading MRSA through indirect contact is by touching objects such as towels, sheets, wound dressings, clothes, counters, door knobs contaminated by the infected skin of a person with MRSA. The spread of MRSA throughout the household is common.

The best way to protect yourself from a MRSA infection is to practice good hygiene. This is done by keeping your hands clean – either by washing them with soap and water or by using an alcohol based hand sanitizer. If your patient has a wound that is draining, or has pus, keep it covered with a clean, dry bandage until it is healed. Be sure your patient understands his healthcare provider's instructions on the proper care of the wound. Pus from infected wounds can contain staph, including MRSA, so keeping the infection covered will help prevent the spread to others including yourself. Bandages and tape from the wound should be put in a bag and discarded with the regular trash. Be sure your patient understands how important it is to not share any personal items with any members of their household. This includes items such as towels, washcloths, razors, clothing or anything that may have had contact with the infected wound or bandage.

You also need to have cleaning procedures for frequently touched surfaces and surfaces that come into direct contact with the skin of your patient.

When caring for someone in their home, it is very important to use "precautions "when caring for them. What do I mean by this? In the medical field we call these precautions standard precautions because they are used in the care of every patient. When following these precautions, all blood, body fluids (except sweat), non- intact skin (open sores) and mucous membranes are treated as if they were infected with an infectious disease. It is important to remember that you cannot tell by looking at someone whether or not they might be infected with something contagious. Referring back to that chain of infection again, using standard precautions will break a link in that chain and therefore stop the spread of the infection.

STANDARD PRECAUTIONS

Standard precautions include:

- Good handwashing
- Wearing gloves if there is a risk of you coming in contact with your patient's bodily fluids, open wounds or mucous membranes
- Wearing a disposable gown to protect your exposed skin and protect soiling of your clothing
- Wearing a mask if you are caring for someone with a respiratory illness.
- Using anti microbial cleaning agents for cleaning surfaces is very important in stopping the spread of infection.

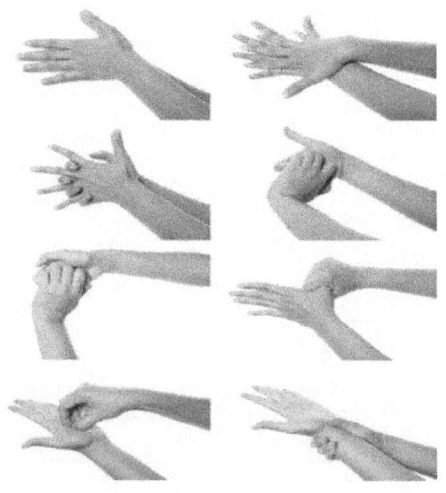

PROPER HANDWASHING TECHNIQUE

Handwashing is the number one way to prevent the spread of infection. The proper handwashing technique includes the following steps:

- Turn on water to a comfortable temperature
- Wet hands and wrists thoroughly
- Apply a generous amount of soap to hands and lather all surfaces of wrists, hands and fingers for 15 to 20 seconds producing friction.
- Clean fingernails by rubbing fingertips against palms of your hands
- Rinse all surfaces of wrists, hands, and fingers. Keep hands pointing down as you rinse. Don't let water run up your arms.
- Use clean, dry paper towels to dry hands completely. Dispose of towels before turning off faucet.
- Use clean, dry paper towel to turn off faucet and then throw away without touching the inside or outside of sink.

ALCOHOL BASED HAND GELS

 Remember that alcohol based hand gels and foams do not take the place of good handwashing. Always use soap and water when your hands are visibly soiled. Also, you should wash your hands when:

- Arriving at your patient's home
- Before handling food or feeding your patient
- After any contact with bodily fluids, contaminated items
- After removing gloves
- Before eating,
- After using the bathroom,
- After blowing your nose or sneezing,
- After smoking
- Before leaving your patients house.

GLOVING AND GOWNING

There is a special order that you need to follow when you put on and take off gloves, gown and mask. The gown goes on first, then the mask and lastly the gloves. When removing this personal protective equipment (PPE), take the dirtiest article off first which are the gloves. Then take the gown off and lastly the mask.

Putting on gloves:

- Wash your hands
- Put on gloves
- Interlace the fingers to smooth out the folds and create a comfortable fit
- Look for tears, holes or discolored spots. Replace gloves if necessary
- If wearing a gown, pull the cuff of the gloves over the sleeve of the gown

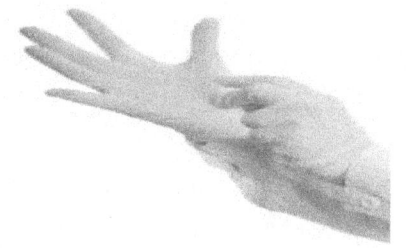

Removing gloves:

- Remove gloves promptly after use and wash your hands
- With one gloved hand, grasp the other glove at the palm, pull the glove off
- Slip fingers from ungloved hand underneath cuff of remaining glove at wrist, and remove glove turning it inside out as it is removed
- Dispose of gloves into designated waste container without contaminating yourself

Putting on gown:

- Pick up gown and unfold it
- Face the back opening of the gown and place arms through each sleeve
- Fasten the neck opening
- Secure gown at waist making sure that the back of your clothing is covered by the gown Make sure the cuff of your gloves overlap the cuffs of your gown

Removing gown:

- After removing gloves, unfasten the gown at the neck and at the waist
- Remove the gown without touching the outside of the gown
- While removing the gown, hold it away from the body and turn it inward and keep it inside out.
- Dispose of the gown in the designated container without contaminating yourself and then wash your hands

Putting on a mask:

- Wash your hands
- Pick up the mask by the top strings or the elastic strap
- Do not touch the mask where it is going to touch your face
- Adjust the mask over your nose and mouth and then tie the top strings first
- If your mask becomes moist, you need to change it

TREATMENT OF MRSA

The treatment for MRSA skin infections may include having a healthcare provider drain the infection and, in some cases, prescribe an antibiotic. **<u>Do not</u>** attempt to treat a MRSA skin infection yourself. This would include popping, draining, or using disinfectants on the area. This could worsen the infection or spread it to others. If you think you or your patient might have an infection, cover the affected skin, wash your hands, and contact a healthcare provider. If an antibiotic is prescribed, be sure to take all of the doses (even if the infection is getting better), unless your healthcare provider tells you to stop taking it. Do not share antibiotics with other people or save unfinished antibiotics to use at another time. If within a few days of visiting your healthcare provider the infection is not getting better, contact him again. If other people you know or live with get the same infection tell them to go to their healthcare provider. It is possible to get repeat infections with MRSA. If you are cured of an infection, you do not become immune to future infections.

MRSA ON HOUSEHOLD SURFACES

MRSA is found on people, but can be transferred from people to inanimate objects by touching infected skin and then touching an object such as a door knob, bed rail, or counter top. If your patient has a skin infection and the wound is not covered, items outside the body can become contaminated by coming in direct contact with the wound. Therefore, it is very important to keep wounds covered with a bandage. If you, the caregiver, touch a surface that has been contaminated with MRSA, it does not mean that you will automatically get an infection. It is, however, important to keep any open areas on your skin covered with a bandage. MRSA can get into the small openings in your skin. Of course, as I have said, the best defense against MRSA is good hand hygiene and wearing disposable gloves if you are dealing with someone's infected wounds.

HOW TO HANDLE SPILLS

Spills involving blood and body fluids can be a serious risk of infection. When blood or body fluids are spilled be sure to put gloves on before cleaning up the spill. If you are cleaning a hard surface such as floor or counter top you can use a solution of one part household bleach to 9 parts of water. You can mix the solution in a container or a plastic spray bottle and then wipe up the spill with rags or paper towels. If the spill is on fabric, you will need to use a commercial disinfectant that does not contain bleach to clean up the spill. If bedding or clothing is soiled, wear gloves and place items in the washing machine. Use color safe bleach along with the detergent to wash the items. Routine laundry procedures, detergents, and laundry additives will all help to make clothes, towels, and linens safe to wear or touch. If items have been contaminated by infectious material, these may be laundered separately, but this is not absolutely necessary.

MRSA AND HOUSEKEEPING

When your patient has a MRSA infection, you need to take special precautions in house cleaning. Disinfectants effective against *Staphylococcus aureus* or staph are most likely also effective against MRSA. These products are readily available from grocery stores and other retail stores. Check the disinfectant product's label on the back of the container. Most, if not all, disinfectant manufacturers will provide a list of germs on their label that their product can destroy. Use disinfectants that are registered by the EPA (check for an EPA registration number on the product's label to confirm that it is registered). Be sure to read the directions on the label too. You will need to know how to safely apply the product to a surface, how long to leave it on the surface, whether or not it needs to be diluted, and most importantly how to keep yourself safe as you use the product.

MRSA AND URINARY TRACT INFECTIONS

If your patient has an indwelling urinary catheter, it is very important to use proper technique in caring for the patient and the catheter so as to help prevent a urinary tract infection. MRSA is a highly contagious organism and if a person has MRSA on one part of the body, it can easily be transferred to another part of the body. In this case, I am referring to the catheter which provides a direct route into the body. If your patient is elderly or has a compromised immune system, this infection can be life threatening. Many elderly patients have contracted MRSA during a hospital or nursing home stay because of the highly contagious nature of MRSA. They have a much harder time fighting off MRSA. Even if your patient does not have a catheter, there is always the risk of them acquiring a UTI especially if your patient is not drinking enough fluids.

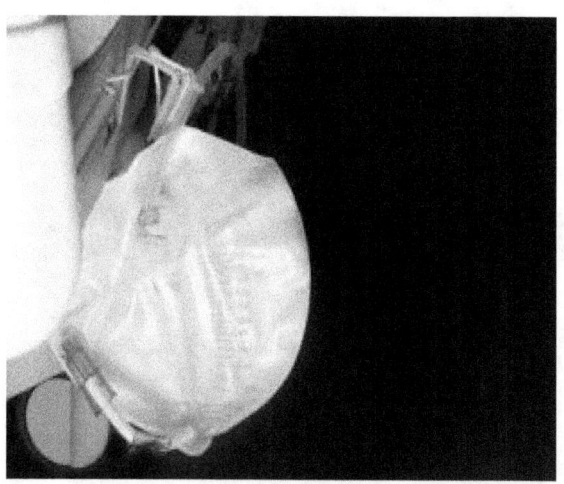

MRSA AND PNEUMONIA

I want to briefly mention how important it is for you to get the flu shot every year. By doing so you can prevent a severe respiratory illness that often follows the flu. Of course, you getting the flu shot can also help to protect your patient against the flu as well. The Pneumonia that can often follow the flu is very often deadly, especially for the older patient. MRSA can affect the respiratory tract and because there is no vaccine against MRSA and the bacterium can live on the skin for a long period of time, MRSA pneumonia is always a risk. MRSA pneumonia is fast-acting and lethal. Once MRSA is inside the body it secrets toxins that eat away the lung tissue. It is a very serious disease which can progress rapidly and is also contagious. Some signs and symptoms of MRSA pneumonia are: cough, sore throat, and head ache, shortness of breath, fever, and chills. If you or your patient should experience any of the respiratory symptoms seek medical help immediately.

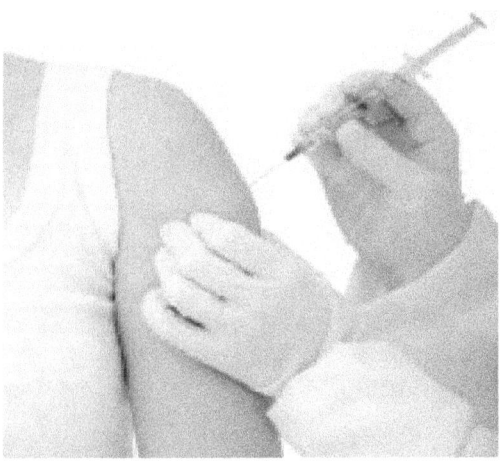

CONCLUSION

I would like to end by saying how important it is to follow all the guidelines that I have outlined in this book in order to prevent a MRSA infection. There is a difference between hospital acquired MRSA infections and community acquired MRSA infections. According to the CDC, the community acquired MRSA is a different strain than the hospital acquired MRSA. The community strain may have some properties that allow it to spread more easily or cause more skin disease. If you suspect a skin infection on yourself or your patient, do not try to treat it yourself. Cover the skin area and seek medical treatment. If you are given an antibiotic, be sure to take it as prescribed. This means taking all of it even if the infection seems better. When your infection is healed, this does not mean that you are now immune to further infections. Therefore, it is important to always follow the guidelines that I have outlined here in order to keep yourself and your patient protected.

RESOURCES

WEBSITES
www.cdc.gov
www.mayoclinic.com

BOOKS
Providing Home Care: A Textbook for Home Health Aides by William Leahy, MD

ABOUT THE AUTHOR

Sharon Kelly is a registered nurse who has a desire to teach caregivers in the home care setting. She has been RN for 30 years and during that time has worked in the fields of Oncology, Infection Control, Education, Home Health and Hospice. To learn more about home caregivers visit Sharon's websites:

www.skillsfornurses.com www.thehomecarer.com

www.ingramcontent.com/pod-product-compliance
Lightning Source LLC
Chambersburg PA
CBHW051423170526
45165CB00004BA/1942